Borrelia burgdorferi

Lyme disease

Constantin Panow

Printed by CreateSpace

"The life so short, the craft so long to learn."

Hippocrates (460-370BC)

Contents

Disclaimer

The author and publisher should not be considered responsible for any deleterious effect, which would result from wrong interpretation and application of following text.

Introduction

This zoonosis is one of most widely distributed diseases in the world.

Endemic areas encompass whole Europe, and huge surfaces of North America and Asia.

It is transmitted by several species of ticks, so called Ixodes parasites.

They need to feed every 3-4 days on a foreign host, and humans are only unintentional victims.

Those insects don't thrive above 2000-2500 m (6500-8200 feet) altitude, and predilection areas are thus prairies and valleys with abundant vegetation.

A lot has been written on the subject, but the reason which stimulated me to participate in this literature, is misunderstanding in the publ c and within professional world as well.

As soon Lyme disease is mentioned, reactions can be neglect, but hysterical exaggeration as well.

Recent title in everyday press, for instance, was: "Is our land still safe for strolling?"

Other illnesses

Besides, ticks are known to transmit also other diseases, at least in Switzerland;

Which are summer meningo- encephalitis, a viral illness, for which there is a vaccination;

And since recently published, Tularemia, (Francisella tularensis), a more serious bacterial ailment.

Borreliosis is recognized since only a few decades. At first it was diagnosed in 1975 in Old Lyme, Connecticut.

It was originally mistaken for other diseases, especially from the rheumatic circle.

Despite better knowledge nowadays, other situations are wrongly interpreted as such.

For instance, a plight which has earned high respect in modernity, fibromyalgia has no true background in my opinion.

As a matter of fact I was able to coin a different diagnosis on every such case admitted with this tag.

For several reasons Borrelia burgdorferi is one of main agents, providing matter for such confusion.

Fibromyalgia

As you can infer from my words I held fibromyalgia for an imposter, a fake disease, invented by self-promoted professors in medicine.

But, as our world is constructed, as we say you need some of everything for it!

If there are lead soldiers, there must be also wooden doctors, for figurative purposes.

The germ involved was first described in 1981 by Willy Burgdorfer.

It is extremely sensitive to most antibiotics.

Despite of this fact, a huge turmoil of ideas still prevails.

People don't understand that most involved population has been exposed to this bacterium since many generations;

Especially as Europeans originate most of the time from Central Asia, an endemic area;

And North Americans- from Europe.

Genuine immune resistance to this disease is present in most people from endemic countries.

Thus, every new infection is encountered with fierce body rejection, and problems occur only in individuals with reduced immunity.

Most of the time this is simply the result of old age and poor general condition, occurring after decades of health neglect, false nutrition and sedentary lifestyle.

Antibiotics

In all other cases healing process is rapid, and thus prescribed antibiotics must catch the sensitive first period of acute inflammation in order to be of any value.

Chronic cases do occur, especially when there is neural involvement.

There are several reasons for this observation, but most important is probably the fact that nerves rely on their own immune system with dedicated cells;

And being seldom pushed to react, they also respond in a more sluggish way.

Coming to diagnosis, essential for early treatment with antibiotics, laboratory exams are pretty disappointing in this direction.

Labs versus clinics

In acute disease, antibodies are present in no more than 50% of cases, which ratio improves with persistence.

Thus, you can as well toss a coin instead.

Not so with the clinical aspect!

You have probably heard about recession of clinical medicine.

There are several reasons for this tendency.

Most important is volume of information, encompassing a huge realm of knowledge from several disciplines.

The other parameter is patient examination, which means you need a valuable degree of sympathy for your neighbor in order to persist in this discipline.

Our society of high modernity, with electronic devices, goes all the opposite way.

Thus, professionals put all their respect in expensive laboratory exams instead of being attentive to what their patient says.

All our modern world goes in a way of individualism,

and people talk less and less to each other.

Thus, the most reliable of all values, a physical examination is relegated to a second degree office.

It takes many years to understand anatomy, and without proficient radiology this is impossible.

How can you transmit to pupils of second year of medicine all knowledge needed for their further exercise of science and profession with only a few lectures and dissections?

Anatomy

Mono-neuritis multiplex is most common involvement with Borreliosis and is readily diagnosed with ultrasound.

It presents as a "string of beads", the nerve being thickened on several places.

Inflammation is not always obvious with Doppler.

Focal thickening exceeds what can be expected with entrapment syndromes, and being multifocal without respecting anatomic boundaries, diagnosis is straightforward.

Here, again, no need to resort to expensive investigative methods.

Meningo- encephalitis, mentioned previously, is an exceptional occurrence.

Skin

But, most common manifestation of disease is cutaneous.

There are three main skin presentations of Lyme disease.

Erythema migrans is present in acute illness, and serology is not obligatory. (As it is seldom positive!)

Lymphocytoma is manifestation of subacute ailment, and serology is positive in 90% of cases.

Acrodermatitis chronica atrophicans is often mistaken for vascular disease, and serology is said to be mandatory for diagnosis, with pretended positivity of 100%.

Uncertainty

This assertion by itself contradicts the basis itself of Science, as there is no method with a sensitivity or reliability of 100%.

The only meaning of this publication, is that involved clinicians didn't have enough experience with diagnosis of acrodermatitis chronica atrophicans on clinical grounds alone.

As a matter of fact, it's a rare condition!

Antibiotic treatment advocated by established medicine for those conditions is respectively of 2, 3 and 4 weeks of doxycycline.

A tick bite has a separate image of a small brownish spot.

Whether due to involved viral or bacterial agents, or chemical-mechanical operation is unknown.

Other germs, as for instance Anaplasma phagocytophilum, are transmitted through tick bites.

Joints

Second most common manifestation of Lyme disease is arthritis.

It presents rather as a low grade synovitis, with tendency to chronicity, in which respect, I advocate antibiotic therapy.

Characteristics are that cartilage is at most thinned.

Synovial reaction is prominent with Doppler hyper-vascularity.

No joint destruction occurs, even after prolonged disease.

No erosions are conspicuous whatsoever.

Other particularity of this condition is rapid healing with antibiotic therapy.

Within 3 days symptoms are completely gone in most cases, which is another way to establish this diagnosis.

Provided, of course, you start treatment in the first two weeks!

Afterwards, in the chronic stage, there is at most slight response.

No point to treat!

Differential diagnosis is in the realm of viral disease, as other bacteria encompass obligatory joint destruction or at least erosive changes.

Many viruses promote a brief arthritic episode.

Few are caught on this evidence, as their result is only fleeted.

Main virus, which can be confused for Borreliosis, is Parvovirus (PVB-19).

Other features peculiar for this disease permit establishment of this diagnosis with certainty.

Pain in this last entity is due to myositis, usually of shoulder region.

Arthritis is said to be of shorter duration than in the case of Lyme disease, but also with reestablishment of whole anatomy without negative results.

Potent clinicians

As you can consider for yourself from previous exposé an informed clinician is very efficient in respect of this illness.

Not every specialty is as well represented.

There is for instance the exception of neurologists, who are still largely unaware of this disease.

One explanation for this fact is their method of investigation.

Main one being EMG, this modality is frequently completely negative in mono-neuritis multiplex.

A "string of beads", because of its anatomy, is completely overlooked by EMG.

Despite huge inflammation, passive electrical transmission remains unchanged.

Probably neural sheath conduction is responsible for this fake.

More on therapy

A peripheral nerve involvement needs one whole week of antibiotic therapy to heal.

Probably owing to lesser penetration of drugs through the neural barrier.

Species

Several species of ticks on those three involved continents transmit Borreliosis.

The ones in Geneva are so tiny, that they are seldom recognized by infested hosts.

One matter, which needs to be exemplified is that aim of the tick is not to be caught on the spot of feeding, but to jump away and go off its prey.

Feeding on its side isn't a suicidal attempt!

Garments

Another deception is that wearing long trousers and socks can prevent tick bites.

Those tiny insects are able to trespass clothing.

Especially summer socks are easy to violate.

Going through the laces makes ticks sometimes tightly caught as in a net, and suffocate.

This is one reason to find them on the skin next morning with clenched mouth-pieces.

Local nursing

Those grabbing hooks can release their contraction on application of a general anesthetic.

Either Ether or Acetone can do the job.

Thus, it is not always necessary to pull and cut.

Gentle application of a cotton swab with the liquid should be sufficient many times.

Of course don't exaggerate!

It is not meant as a race between the animal and you to see who would fall asleep first.

Surgical action can help in resilient cases.

To come back to fibromyalgia, I must admit that not everything is known about Lyme disease.

For instance, some cases of Reiter's syndrome are possibly related to this entity.

Among gardeners it is said that ticks jump and fall from trees.

Thus, if you want a whole body protection, even a burqa wouldn't do the job!

But, as I told you at the beginning of this small publication, we are endowed with a good immunity from Mother Nature.

In this respect, probably only a small percentage of cases come to medical attention whatsoever.

Most Borreliosis infections heal unrecognized and untreated.

Website

I hope you enjoyed this short publication.

For any comment or if you have questions you can reach me at:

www.thenopillshealthprospect.com

If so, don't hesitate!

Write in my blog!